The Essential Foods Lists For Kidney Disease

Curated Dietary Selections for Optimal Renal Health, Empower yourself with dietary choices and promoting your well being

Anita Hulsey

Table of Contents

INTRODUCTION

Meet Simon, a lively and energetic individual who has always enjoyed the simple pleasures of life, from morning jogs to cooking delicious meals for his family. Recently, Simon was diagnosed with chronic kidney disease (CKD), a condition that necessitated significant changes to his lifestyle, particularly his diet. Initially overwhelmed by the dietary restrictions and the abundance of conflicting information, Simon embarked on a journey to discover the essential foods that would support his kidney health without sacrificing flavor and enjoyment.

Through diligent research and consulting with nutritionists, Simon learned that a kidney-friendly diet isn't just about cutting out certain foods, but also about embracing a variety of nutrient-rich options that cater to his new needs. He discovered the importance of balancing essential nutrients, managing sodium intake, and choosing the right proteins, all while still enjoying satisfying and tasty meals.

In this guide, The Essential Foods Lists For Kidney Disease, Simon shares his insights and experiences, aiming to help others navigate their dietary journey with ease. From understanding which foods to prioritize to finding joy in cooking kidney-friendly recipes, Simon's story is a testament to the power of informed choices and a positive mindset. Join Simon as he explores a comprehensive list of essential foods and shares delicious recipes for breakfast, lunch, and dinner, making the path to better kidney health both attainable and enjoyable.

CHAPTER ONE

Breakfast Recipes

- Blueberry Oatmeal

Blueberry Oatmeal Recipes

Recipe 1:

Classic Blueberry Oatmeal

Ingredients:
- 1 cup rolled oats
- 2 cups water or low-fat milk
- 1 cup fresh or frozen blueberries
- 1 tablespoon honey or maple syrup (optional)
- 1/2 teaspoon vanilla extract
- A pinch of salt

- 1/4 teaspoon ground cinnamon (optional)

Instructions:
1. In a medium saucepan, bring water or milk to a boil.
2. Add oats and a pinch of salt, then reduce heat to medium-low.
3. Cook, stirring occasionally, until the oats are tender and the mixture is creamy, about 5-7 minutes.
4. Stir in blueberries, honey or maple syrup, vanilla extract, and cinnamon.
5. Cook for another 2-3 minutes until blueberries are softened.
6. Serve warm, optionally topped with a few extra blueberries and a drizzle of honey.

Nutritional Information (per serving):
- Calories: 210
- Protein: 6g
- Carbohydrates: 45g
- Dietary Fiber: 6g
- Sugars: 10g

- Fat: 3g
- Sodium: 60mg

Cooking Time:10 minutes
Serving Size:2 servings

Recipe 2:

Blueberry Almond Oatmeal

Ingredients:
- 1 cup rolled oats
- 2 cups almond milk
- 1 cup fresh or frozen blueberries
- 2 tablespoons almond butter
- 1 tablespoon honey or agave syrup
- 1/2 teaspoon vanilla extract
- A pinch of salt
- 1/4 cup sliced almonds (optional)

Instructions:
1. In a medium saucepan, bring almond milk to a boil.
2. Add oats and a pinch of salt, then reduce heat to medium-low.

3. Cook, stirring occasionally, until the oats are tender and the mixture is creamy, about 5-7 minutes.
4. Stir in blueberries, almond butter, honey or agave syrup, and vanilla extract.
5. Cook for another 2-3 minutes until blueberries are softened.
6. Serve warm, topped with sliced almonds.

Nutritional Information (per serving):
- Calories: 250
- Protein: 8g
- Carbohydrates: 45g
- Dietary Fiber: 7g
- Sugars: 12g
- Fat: 8g
- Sodium: 70mg

Cooking Time:10 minutes
Serving Size: 2 servings

Recipe 3:

Blueberry Banana Oatmeal

Ingredients:
- 1 cup rolled oats
- 2 cups water or low-fat milk
- 1 cup fresh or frozen blueberries
- 1 ripe banana, sliced
- 1 tablespoon honey or maple syrup (optional)
- 1/2 teaspoon vanilla extract
- A pinch of salt
- 1/4 teaspoon ground cinnamon (optional)

Instructions:
1. In a medium saucepan, bring water or milk to a boil.
2. Add oats and a pinch of salt, then reduce heat to medium-low.
3. Cook, stirring occasionally, until the oats are tender and the mixture is creamy, about 5-7 minutes.

4. Stir in blueberries, banana slices, honey or maple syrup, vanilla extract, and cinnamon.
5. Cook for another 2-3 minutes until blueberries are softened.
6. Serve warm, optionally topped with extra banana slices and blueberries.

Nutritional Information (per serving):
- Calories: 230
- Protein: 5g
- Carbohydrates: 50g
- Dietary Fiber: 7g
- Sugars: 15g
- Fat: 3g
- Sodium: 60mg

Cooking Time:10 minutes
Serving Size: 2 servings

Recipe 4:

Blueberry Walnut Oatmeal

Ingredients:

- 1 cup rolled oats
- 2 cups water or low-fat milk
- 1 cup fresh or frozen blueberries
- 2 tablespoons chopped walnuts
- 1 tablespoon honey or maple syrup (optional)
- 1/2 teaspoon vanilla extract
- A pinch of salt
- 1/4 teaspoon ground cinnamon (optional)

Instructions:

1. In a medium saucepan, bring water or milk to a boil.

2. Add oats and a pinch of salt, then reduce heat to medium-low.

3. Cook, stirring occasionally, until the oats are tender and the mixture is creamy, about 5-7 minutes.

4. Stir in blueberries, chopped walnuts, honey or maple syrup, vanilla extract, and cinnamon.

5. Cook for another 2-3 minutes until blueberries are softened.

6. Serve warm, optionally topped with extra chopped walnuts and blueberries.

Nutritional Information (per serving):
- Calories: 240
- Protein: 6g
- Carbohydrates: 45g
- Dietary Fiber: 6g
- Sugars: 10g
- Fat: 7g
- Sodium: 60mg

Cooking Time: 10 minutes
Serving Size: 2 servings

- Veggie Egg White Omelette

Recipe 1:

Spinach and Feta Egg White Omelette

Ingredients:
- 4 egg whites
- 1/4 cup fresh spinach, chopped
- 2 tbsp crumbled feta cheese
- 1 tbsp minced onion
- 1 tsp olive oil
- Salt and pepper to taste

Nutritional Information (per serving):
- Calories: 110
- Protein: 15g
- Fat: 4g
- Carbs: 4g

Cooking Time: 10 minutes
Serving Size: 1 omelette

Instructions:
1. Beat the egg whites in a bowl until frothy.
2. Heat the olive oil in a non-stick pan over medium heat.
3. Add the minced onion and sauté for 2-3 minutes until translucent.

4. Add the chopped spinach and sauté for another minute.

5. Pour the egg whites into the pan and let them cook for 2-3 minutes.

6. Sprinkle the feta cheese over the top of the omelette.

7. Fold the omelette in half and cook for an additional 2-3 minutes.

8. Slide the omelette onto a plate and season with salt and pepper.

Recipe 2:

Veggie Medley Egg White Omelette

Ingredients:
- 4 egg whites
- 1/4 cup diced bell pepper
- 1/4 cup diced mushrooms
- 2 tbsp diced tomatoes
- 1 tbsp minced garlic
- 1 tsp olive oil
- Salt and pepper to taste

Nutritional Information (per serving):

- Calories: 100
- Protein: 16g
- Fat: 3g
- Carbs: 5g

Cooking Time: 12 minutes
Serving Size: 1 omelette

Instructions:
1. Beat the egg whites in a bowl until frothy.
2. Heat the olive oil in a non-stick pan over medium heat.
3. Add the minced garlic and sauté for 1 minute.
4. Add the diced bell pepper, mushrooms, and tomatoes to the pan and sauté for 3-4 minutes.
5. Pour the egg whites into the pan and let them cook for 3-4 minutes.
6. Using a spatula, gently fold the omelette in half.
7. Cook for an additional 2-3 minutes.
8. Slide the omelette onto a plate and season with salt and pepper.

Recipe 3:

 Asparagus and Cheese Egg White Omelette

Ingredients:
- 4 egg whites
- 1/4 cup chopped asparagus
- 2 tbsp shredded cheddar cheese
- 1 tbsp minced onion
- 1 tsp olive oil
- Salt and pepper to taste

Nutritional Information (per serving):
- Calories: 120
- Protein: 15g
- Fat: 5g
- Carbs: 3g

Cooking Time: 12 minutes
Serving Size: 1 omelette

Instructions:

1. Beat the egg whites in a bowl until frothy.
2. Heat the olive oil in a non-stick pan over medium heat.
3. Add the minced onion and sauté for 2-3 minutes until translucent.
4. Add the chopped asparagus to the pan and sauté for 3-4 minutes.
5. Pour the egg whites into the pan and let them cook for 3-4 minutes.
6. Sprinkle the shredded cheddar cheese over the top of the omelette.
7. Fold the omelette in half and cook for an additional 2-3 minutes.
8. Slide the omelette onto a plate and season with salt and pepper.

Recipe 4:

Broccoli and Tomato Egg White Omelette

Ingredients:
- 4 egg whites
- 1/4 cup chopped broccoli
- 2 tbsp diced tomatoes

- 1 tbsp minced red onion
- 1 tsp olive oil
- Salt and pepper to taste

Nutritional Information (per serving):
- Calories: 100
- Protein: 16g
- Fat: 3g
- Carbs: 4g

Cooking Time: 12 minutes
Serving Size: 1 omelette

Instructions:
1. Beat the egg whites in a bowl until frothy.
2. Heat the olive oil in a non-stick pan over medium heat.
3. Add the minced red onion and sauté for 2-3 minutes.
4. Add the chopped broccoli to the pan and sauté for 3-4 minutes.
5. Add the diced tomatoes and sauté for another minute.

6. Pour the egg whites into the pan and let them cook for 3-4 minutes.

7. Using a spatula, gently fold the omelette in half.

8. Cook for an additional 2-3 minutes.

9. Slide the omelette onto a plate and season with salt and pepper.

- Kidney-Friendly Smoothie

Recipe 1:

Blueberry Banana Kidney-Friendly Smoothie

Ingredients:
- 1 cup unsweetened almond milk
- 1/2 cup fresh or frozen blueberries
- 1 small ripe banana
- 1 tbsp ground flaxseed
- 1 tsp honey (optional)

Nutritional Information (per serving):

- Calories: 180
- Protein: 4g
- Fat: 6g
- Carbs: 28g
- Potassium: 350mg
- Phosphorus: 125mg

Cooking Time: 5 minutes
Serving Size: 1 smoothie

Instructions:
1. Add all the ingredients to a blender.
2. Blend on high speed until smooth and creamy.
3. Pour the smoothie into a glass and enjoy.

Recipe 2:

Kiwi Pineapple Kidney-Friendly Smoothie

Ingredients:
- 1 cup unsweetened coconut milk
- 1 kiwi, peeled and chopped
- 1/2 cup fresh or frozen pineapple chunks

- 1 tbsp chia seeds
- 1 tsp honey (optional)

Nutritional Information (per serving):
- Calories: 190
- Protein: 3g
- Fat: 10g
- Carbs: 22g
- Potassium: 330mg
- Phosphorus: 115mg

Cooking Time: 5 minutes
Serving Size: 1 smoothie

Instructions:
1. Add all the ingredients to a blender.
2. Blend on high speed until smooth and creamy.
3. Pour the smoothie into a glass and enjoy.

Recipe 3:

Mango Peach Kidney-Friendly Smoothie

Ingredients:
- 1 cup unsweetened almond milk
- 1/2 cup fresh or frozen mango chunks
- 1/2 cup fresh or frozen peach slices
- 1 tbsp unsweetened shredded coconut
- 1 tsp lime juice

Nutritional Information (per serving):
- Calories: 170
- Protein: 3g
- Fat: 5g
- Carbs: 28g
- Potassium: 350mg
- Phosphorus: 100mg

Cooking Time: 5 minutes
Serving Size: 1 smoothie

Instructions:
1. Add all the ingredients to a blender.
2. Blend on high speed until smooth and creamy.
3. Pour the smoothie into a glass and enjoy.

Recipe 4:

Strawberry Avocado Kidney-Friendly Smoothie

Ingredients:
- 1 cup unsweetened coconut milk
- 1/2 cup fresh or frozen strawberries
- 1/4 ripe avocado
- 1 tbsp almond butter
- 1 tsp honey (optional)

Nutritional Information (per serving):
- Calories: 240
- Protein: 5g
- Fat: 15g
- Carbs: 20g
- Potassium: 380mg
- Phosphorus: 140mg

Cooking Time: 5 minutes
Serving Size: 1 smoothie

Instructions:
1. Add all the ingredients to a blender.

2. Blend on high speed until smooth and creamy.

3. Pour the smoothie into a glass and enjoy.

- Quinoa Breakfast Bowl

Recipe 1:

Blueberry Quinoa Breakfast Bowl

Ingredients:
- 1/2 cup cooked quinoa
- 1/2 cup fresh or frozen blueberries
- 2 tbsp unsweetened almond milk
- 1 tsp honey
- 1 tbsp sliced almonds
- 1 tsp chia seeds

Nutritional Information (per serving):
- Calories: 240
- Protein: 8g
- Fat: 9g
- Carbs: 35g

- Fiber: 6g
- Potassium: 300mg
- Phosphorus: 200mg

Cooking Time: 10 minutes
Serving Size: 1 bowl

Instructions:
1. Cook the quinoa according to package instructions.
2. In a bowl, combine the cooked quinoa, blueberries, almond milk, and honey.
3. Top with sliced almonds and chia seeds.
4. Enjoy your Blueberry Quinoa Breakfast Bowl!

Recipe 2:

Apple Cinnamon Quinoa Breakfast Bowl

Ingredients:
- 1/2 cup cooked quinoa
- 1/2 cup diced apple
- 2 tbsp unsweetened almond milk
- 1 tsp cinnamon

- 1 tbsp chopped walnuts
- 1 tsp maple syrup (optional)

Nutritional Information (per serving):
- Calories: 255
- Protein: 7g
- Fat: 11g
- Carbs: 35g
- Fiber: 5g
- Potassium: 280mg
- Phosphorus: 220mg

Cooking Time: 10 minutes
Serving Size: 1 bowl

Instructions:
1. Cook the quinoa according to package instructions.
2. In a bowl, combine the cooked quinoa, diced apple, almond milk, and cinnamon.
3. Top with chopped walnuts and drizzle with maple syrup (if using).
4. Enjoy your Apple Cinnamon Quinoa Breakfast Bowl!

Recipe 3:

Tropical Quinoa Breakfast Bowl

Ingredients:
- 1/2 cup cooked quinoa
- 1/2 cup diced pineapple
- 1/4 cup diced mango
- 2 tbsp unsweetened coconut milk
- 1 tbsp shredded coconut
- 1 tsp lime juice

Nutritional Information (per serving):
- Calories: 265
- Protein: 6g
- Fat: 10g
- Carbs: 40g
- Fiber: 5g
- Potassium: 350mg
- Phosphorus: 180mg

Cooking Time: 10 minutes
Serving Size: 1 bowl

Instructions:

1. Cook the quinoa according to package instructions.
2. In a bowl, combine the cooked quinoa, diced pineapple, diced mango, and coconut milk.
3. Top with shredded coconut and a drizzle of lime juice.
4. Enjoy your Tropical Quinoa Breakfast Bowl!

Recipe 4:

Savory Quinoa Breakfast Bowl

Ingredients:
- 1/2 cup cooked quinoa
- 1 poached egg
- 2 tbsp diced avocado
- 1 tbsp diced tomato
- 1 tbsp crumbled feta cheese
- 1 tsp chopped fresh basil
- 1 tbsp olive oil
- Salt and pepper to taste

Nutritional Information (per serving):

- Calories: 280
- Protein: 12g
- Fat: 15g
- Carbs: 25g
- Fiber: 5g
- Potassium: 400mg
- Phosphorus: 250mg

Cooking Time: 15 minutes
Serving Size: 1 bowl

Instructions:
1. Cook the quinoa according to package instructions.
2. Poach an egg according to your preferred method.
3. In a bowl, combine the cooked quinoa, poached egg, diced avocado, diced tomato, crumbled feta cheese, and chopped fresh basil.
4. Drizzle with olive oil and season with salt and pepper.
5. Enjoy your Savory Quinoa Breakfast Bowl!

CHAPTER TWO

Lunch Recipes

- Grilled Chicken Salad with Low-Sodium Dressing

Recipe 1:

Mediterranean Grilled Chicken Salad with Lemon-Herb Dressing

Ingredients:
- 4 oz grilled chicken breast, sliced
- 2 cups mixed greens
- 1/4 cup diced cucumber
- 1/4 cup diced tomato
- 2 tbsp crumbled feta cheese
- 1 tbsp sliced kalamata olives
- 2 tbsp lemon-herb dressing (see recipe below)

Lemon-Herb Dressing:
- 2 tbsp olive oil
- 1 tbsp lemon juice
- 1 tsp Dijon mustard
- 1 tsp chopped fresh herbs (e.g., parsley, basil, oregano)
- 1/4 tsp garlic powder
- 1/8 tsp salt
- 1/8 tsp black pepper

Nutritional Information (per serving):
- Calories: 280
- Protein: 28g
- Fat: 15g
- Carbs: 10g
- Fiber: 4g
- Sodium: 330mg

Cooking Time: 15 minutes
Serving Size: 1 salad

Instructions:

1. Prepare the lemon-herb dressing by mixing all the dressing ingredients in a small bowl.
2. Grill the chicken breast until cooked through, then slice it.
3. In a large bowl, combine the mixed greens, diced cucumber, diced tomato, feta cheese, and sliced olives.
4. Top the salad with the grilled chicken slices and drizzle the lemon-herb dressing over the top.
5. Enjoy your Mediterranean Grilled Chicken Salad!

Recipe 2:

 Southwest Grilled Chicken Salad with Avocado-Lime Dressing

Ingredients:
- 4 oz grilled chicken breast, sliced
- 2 cups mixed greens
- 1/4 cup diced bell pepper
- 1/4 cup diced red onion
- 2 tbsp diced avocado

- 1 tbsp roasted corn kernels
- 2 tbsp avocado-lime dressing (see recipe below)

Avocado-Lime Dressing:
- 1/2 avocado
- 2 tbsp lime juice
- 1 tbsp olive oil
- 1/4 tsp garlic powder
- 1/8 tsp salt
- 1/8 tsp black pepper

Nutritional Information (per serving):
- Calories: 290
- Protein: 29g
- Fat: 16g
- Carbs: 12g
- Fiber: 5g
- Sodium: 310mg

Cooking Time: 15 minutes
Serving Size: 1 salad

Instructions:

1. Prepare the avocado-lime dressing by blending all the dressing ingredients in a food processor or blender until smooth.
2. Grill the chicken breast until cooked through, then slice it.
3. In a large bowl, combine the mixed greens, diced bell pepper, diced red onion, diced avocado, and roasted corn kernels.
4. Top the salad with the grilled chicken slices and drizzle the avocado-lime dressing over the top.
5. Enjoy your Southwest Grilled Chicken Salad!

Recipe 3:

Asian Grilled Chicken Salad with Sesame-Ginger Dressing

Ingredients:
- 4 oz grilled chicken breast, sliced
- 2 cups mixed greens
- 1/4 cup shredded carrots
- 1/4 cup diced cucumber
- 1 tbsp toasted sesame seeds

- 2 tbsp sesame-ginger dressing (see recipe below)

Sesame-Ginger Dressing:
- 2 tbsp rice vinegar
- 1 tbsp low-sodium soy sauce
- 1 tsp sesame oil
- 1 tsp grated ginger
- 1/4 tsp garlic powder
- 1/8 tsp salt
- 1/8 tsp black pepper

Nutritional Information (per serving):
- Calories: 260
- Protein: 27g
- Fat: 12g
- Carbs: 13g
- Fiber: 3g
- Sodium: 350mg

Cooking Time: 15 minutes
Serving Size: 1 salad

Instructions:

1. Prepare the sesame-ginger dressing by whisking all the dressing ingredients in a small bowl.
2. Grill the chicken breast until cooked through, then slice it.
3. In a large bowl, combine the mixed greens, shredded carrots, and diced cucumber.
4. Top the salad with the grilled chicken slices and sprinkle the toasted sesame seeds over the top.
5. Drizzle the sesame-ginger dressing over the salad.
6. Enjoy your Asian Grilled Chicken Salad!

Recipe 4:

Cobb Grilled Chicken Salad with Buttermilk Ranch Dressing

Ingredients:
- 4 oz grilled chicken breast, sliced
- 2 cups mixed greens
- 1 hard-boiled egg, sliced
- 2 tbsp crumbled blue cheese

- 2 tbsp diced tomato
- 2 tbsp diced avocado
- 2 tbsp buttermilk ranch dressing (see recipe below)

Buttermilk Ranch Dressing:
- 1/4 cup low-fat buttermilk
- 2 tbsp plain Greek yogurt
- 1 tbsp chopped fresh parsley
- 1 tsp lemon juice
- 1/4 tsp garlic powder
- 1/8 tsp salt
- 1/8 tsp black pepper

Nutritional Information (per serving):
- Calories: 280
- Protein: 27g
- Fat: 15g
- Carbs: 10g
- Fiber: 4g
- Sodium: 370mg

Cooking Time: 15 minutes
Serving Size: 1 salad

Instructions:
1. Prepare the buttermilk ranch dressing by mixing all the dressing ingredients in a small bowl.
2. Grill the chicken breast until cooked through, then slice it.
3. In a large bowl, combine the mixed greens, sliced hard-boiled egg, crumbled blue cheese, diced tomato, and diced avocado.
4. Top the salad with the grilled chicken slices and drizzle the buttermilk ranch dressing over the top.
5. Enjoy your Cobb Grilled Chicken Salad!

   - Turkey and Avocado Wrap

Recipe 1: Roasted Turkey and Avocado Wrap

Ingredients:
- 4 oz roasted turkey breast, sliced
- 1/2 avocado, sliced

- 2 tbsp shredded lettuce
- 1 tbsp diced tomato
- 1 tbsp low-fat mayonnaise
- 1 tsp Dijon mustard
- 1 whole-wheat tortilla or wrap

Nutritional Information (per serving):
- Calories: 320
- Protein: 24g
- Fat: 16g
- Carbs: 25g
- Fiber: 7g
- Sodium: 650mg

Cooking Time: 10 minutes
Serving Size: 1 wrap

Instructions:
1. Spread the low-fat mayonnaise and Dijon mustard on the whole-wheat tortilla or wrap.
2. Layer the roasted turkey slices, avocado slices, shredded lettuce, and diced tomato on the tortilla.

3. Carefully roll up the tortilla to enclose the filling.
4. Serve the Roasted Turkey and Avocado Wrap immediately.

Recipe 2: Smoked Turkey and Avocado Wrap

Ingredients:
- 4 oz smoked turkey breast, sliced
- 1/2 avocado, mashed
- 2 tbsp chopped red onion
- 1 tbsp chopped fresh cilantro
- 1 tbsp low-fat sour cream
- 1 tsp lime juice
- 1 whole-wheat tortilla or wrap

Nutritional Information (per serving):
- Calories: 330
- Protein: 25g
- Fat: 17g
- Carbs: 26g
- Fiber: 6g
- Sodium: 670mg

Cooking Time: 10 minutes
Serving Size: 1 wrap

Instructions:
1. In a small bowl, mash the avocado and mix in the chopped red onion, fresh cilantro, low-fat sour cream, and lime juice.
2. Spread the avocado mixture on the whole-wheat tortilla or wrap.
3. Layer the smoked turkey slices on top of the avocado mixture.
4. Carefully roll up the tortilla to enclose the filling.
5. Serve the Smoked Turkey and Avocado Wrap immediately.

Recipe 3: Honey Mustard Turkey and Avocado Wrap

Ingredients:
- 4 oz roasted turkey breast, sliced
- 1/2 avocado, sliced
- 2 tbsp shredded carrots
- 1 tbsp honey mustard dressing

- 1 whole-wheat tortilla or wrap

Nutritional Information (per serving):
- Calories: 310
- Protein: 23g
- Fat: 15g
- Carbs: 27g
- Fiber: 6g
- Sodium: 580mg

Cooking Time: 10 minutes
Serving Size: 1 wrap

Instructions:
1. Spread the honey mustard dressing on the whole-wheat tortilla or wrap.
2. Layer the roasted turkey slices, avocado slices, and shredded carrots on the tortilla.
3. Carefully roll up the tortilla to enclose the filling.
4. Serve the Honey Mustard Turkey and Avocado Wrap immediately.

Recipe 4: Chipotle Turkey and Avocado Wrap

Ingredients:
- 4 oz roasted turkey breast, sliced
- 1/2 avocado, mashed
- 2 tbsp diced tomato
- 1 tbsp chopped fresh cilantro
- 1 tsp chipotle sauce or paste
- 1 whole-wheat tortilla or wrap

Nutritional Information (per serving):
- Calories: 330
- Protein: 24g
- Fat: 16g
- Carbs: 28g
- Fiber: 7g
- Sodium: 620mg

Cooking Time: 10 minutes
Serving Size: 1 wrap

Instructions:
1. In a small bowl, mash the avocado and mix in the diced tomato, chopped fresh cilantro, and chipotle sauce or paste.

2. Spread the avocado mixture on the whole-wheat tortilla or wrap.

3. Layer the roasted turkey slices on top of the avocado mixture.

4. Carefully roll up the tortilla to enclose the filling.

5. Serve the Chipotle Turkey and Avocado Wrap immediately.

- Lentil and Veggie Soup

Recipe 1:

Classic Lentil and Veggie Soup

Ingredients:
- 1 cup dried brown lentils, rinsed
- 4 cups low-sodium vegetable broth
- 1 tbsp olive oil
- 1 onion, diced
- 2 carrots, peeled and diced
- 2 celery stalks, diced
- 3 garlic cloves, minced

- 1 tsp ground cumin
- 1 tsp dried oregano
- 1/4 tsp crushed red pepper flakes (optional)
- Salt and black pepper to taste
- 2 cups chopped kale or spinach

Nutritional Information (per serving):
- Calories: 240
- Protein: 14g
- Fat: 5g
- Carbs: 37g
- Fiber: 12g
- Sodium: 420mg

Cooking Time: 45 minutes
Serving Size: 1 cup

Instructions:
1. In a large pot, bring the vegetable broth to a boil over high heat. Add the lentils, reduce heat to medium-low, and simmer for 20-25 minutes, or until the lentils are tender.

2. In a separate skillet, heat the olive oil over medium heat. Add the onion, carrots, and celery, and sauté for about 5 minutes, or until the vegetables are softened.
3. Add the garlic, cumin, oregano, and red pepper flakes (if using) to the skillet. Sauté for 1 minute, or until fragrant.
4. Transfer the sautéed vegetables to the pot with the cooked lentils. Season with salt and black pepper to taste.
5. Add the chopped kale or spinach and simmer for an additional 5-10 minutes, or until the greens are wilted.
6. Serve the Classic Lentil and Veggie Soup hot.

Recipe 2:

 Curried Lentil and Veggie Soup

Ingredients:
- 1 cup dried red lentils, rinsed
- 4 cups low-sodium vegetable broth
- 1 tbsp olive oil
- 1 onion, diced

- 2 garlic cloves, minced
- 1 tbsp grated fresh ginger
- 2 tsp curry powder
- 1 tsp ground cumin
- 1/4 tsp cayenne pepper (optional)
- 1 cup diced sweet potatoes
- 1 cup diced cauliflower florets
- Salt and black pepper to taste
- 2 tbsp chopped fresh cilantro (for garnish)

Nutritional Information (per serving):
- Calories: 260
- Protein: 13g
- Fat: 6g
- Carbs: 39g
- Fiber: 11g
- Sodium: 380mg

Cooking Time: 40 minutes
Serving Size: 1 cup

Instructions:
1. In a large pot, bring the vegetable broth to a boil over high heat. Add the red

lentils, reduce heat to medium-low, and simmer for 15-20 minutes, or until the lentils are tender.
2. In a separate skillet, heat the olive oil over medium heat. Add the onion and sauté for 3-4 minutes, or until translucent.
3. Add the garlic, grated ginger, curry powder, cumin, and cayenne pepper (if using) to the skillet. Sauté for 1 minute, or until fragrant.
4. Transfer the sautéed aromatics to the pot with the cooked lentils. Add the diced sweet potatoes and cauliflower florets.
5. Simmer the soup for an additional 15-20 minutes, or until the vegetables are tender.
6. Season the Curried Lentil and Veggie Soup with salt and black pepper to taste.
7. Serve the soup hot, garnished with chopped fresh cilantro.

Recipe 3:

Tuscan Lentil and Veggie Soup

Ingredients:

- 1 cup dried green or brown lentils, rinsed
- 4 cups low-sodium vegetable broth
- 1 tbsp olive oil
- 1 onion, diced
- 2 carrots, peeled and diced
- 2 celery stalks, diced
- 3 garlic cloves, minced
- 1 tsp dried thyme
- 1 tsp dried basil
- 1 (14.5 oz) can diced tomatoes
- 1 cup chopped kale or spinach
- Salt and black pepper to taste
- Grated Parmesan cheese for serving (optional)

Nutritional Information (per serving):
- Calories: 270
- Protein: 15g
- Fat: 6g
- Carbs: 40g
- Fiber: 13g
- Sodium: 460mg

Cooking Time: 45 minutes
Serving Size: 1 cup

Instructions:

1. In a large pot, bring the vegetable broth to a boil over high heat. Add the lentils, reduce heat to medium-low, and simmer for 20-25 minutes, or until the lentils are tender.

2. In a separate skillet, heat the olive oil over medium heat. Add the onion, carrots, and celery, and sauté for about 5 minutes, or until the vegetables are softened.

3. Add the garlic, dried thyme, and dried basil to the skillet. Sauté for 1 minute, or until fragrant.

4. Transfer the sautéed vegetables to the pot with the cooked lentils. Add the diced tomatoes and their juices.

5. Simmer the Tuscan Lentil and Veggie Soup for an additional 10-15 minutes, or until the vegetables are tender.

6. Stir in the chopped kale or spinach and season with salt and black pepper to taste.

7. Serve the soup hot, garnished with grated Parmesan cheese (if desired).

Recipe 4:

Hearty Lentil and Vegetable Soup

Ingredients:
- 1 cup dried brown lentils, rinsed
- 4 cups low-sodium vegetable broth
- 1 tbsp olive oil
- 1 onion, diced
- 2 carrots, peeled and diced
- 2 celery stalks, diced
- 3 garlic cloves, minced
- 1 tsp dried oregano
- 1 tsp dried basil
- 1 (15 oz) can diced tomatoes
- 1 cup frozen mixed vegetables (such as peas, corn, and green beans)
- Salt and black pepper to taste
- Chopped fresh parsley for garnish (optional)

Nutritional Information (per serving):
- Calories: 280
- Protein: 15g
- Fat: 6g

- Carbs: 41g
- Fiber: 12g
- Sodium: 430mg

Cooking Time: 45 minutes
Serving Size: 1 cup

Instructions:
1. In a large pot, bring the vegetable broth to a boil over high heat. Add the lentils, reduce heat to medium-low, and simmer for 20-25 minutes, or until the lentils are tender.
2. In a separate skillet, heat the olive oil over medium heat. Add the onion, carrots, and celery, and sauté for about 5 minutes, or until the vegetables are softened.
3. Add the garlic, dried oregano, and dried basil to the skillet. Sauté for 1 minute, or until fragrant.
4. Transfer the sautéed vegetables to the pot with the cooked lentils. Add the diced tomatoes and their juices, as well as the frozen mixed vegetables.

5. Simmer the Hearty Lentil and Vegetable Soup for an additional 10-15 minutes, or until the vegetables are tender.
6. Season the soup with salt and black pepper to taste.
7. Serve the soup hot, garnished with chopped fresh parsley (if desired).

- Quinoa and Black Bean Salad

Recipe 1:

Zesty Quinoa and Black Bean Salad

Ingredients:
- 1 cup quinoa, rinsed
- 1 (15oz) can black beans, drained and rinsed
- 1 cup diced bell pepper (mix of red, yellow, and/or orange)
- 1/2 cup diced red onion
- 1/4 cup chopped fresh cilantro

- 2 tablespoons lime juice
- 2 tablespoons olive oil
- 1 teaspoon ground cumin
- 1/2 teaspoon salt
- 1/4 teaspoon black pepper

Nutrition (per serving):
Calories: 255, Total Fat: 8g, Saturated Fat: 1g, Sodium: 330mg, Carbohydrates: 37g, Fiber: 8g, Protein: 9g

Cooking Time: 20 minutes
Serves: 4

Instructions:
1. Cook quinoa according to package instructions. Allow to cool slightly.
2. In a large bowl, combine the cooked quinoa, black beans, bell pepper, red onion, and cilantro.
3. In a small bowl, whisk together the lime juice, olive oil, cumin, salt, and black pepper.
4. Pour the dressing over the quinoa mixture and toss gently to combine.

5. Serve chilled or at room temperature.

Recipe 2:

 Southwestern Quinoa and Black Bean Salad

Ingredients:
- 1 cup quinoa, rinsed
- 1 (15oz) can black beans, drained and rinsed
- 1 cup corn kernels (fresh or frozen)
- 1/2 cup diced tomatoes
- 1/4 cup chopped green onions
- 2 tablespoons chopped fresh cilantro
- 2 tablespoons lime juice
- 1 tablespoon olive oil
- 1 teaspoon chili powder
- 1/2 teaspoon ground cumin
- 1/4 teaspoon salt

Nutrition (per serving):
Calories: 270, Total Fat: 7g, Saturated Fat: 1g, Sodium: 350mg, Carbohydrates: 42g, Fiber: 9g, Protein: 10g

Cooking Time: 20 minutes
Serves: 4

Instructions:
1. Cook quinoa according to package instructions. Allow to cool slightly.
2. In a large bowl, combine the cooked quinoa, black beans, corn, tomatoes, green onions, and cilantro.
3. In a small bowl, whisk together the lime juice, olive oil, chili powder, cumin, and salt.
4. Pour the dressing over the quinoa mixture and toss gently to combine.
5. Serve chilled or at room temperature.

Recipe 3:

 Mediterranean Quinoa and Black Bean Salad

Ingredients:
- 1 cup quinoa, rinsed

- 1 (15oz) can black beans, drained and rinsed
- 1/2 cup diced cucumber
- 1/2 cup crumbled feta cheese
- 1/4 cup chopped kalamata olives
- 2 tablespoons chopped fresh parsley
- 2 tablespoons lemon juice
- 1 tablespoon olive oil
- 1 teaspoon dried oregano
- 1/4 teaspoon salt
- 1/4 teaspoon black pepper

Nutrition (per serving):
Calories: 265, Total Fat: 10g, Saturated Fat: 3g, Sodium: 375mg, Carbohydrates: 33g, Fiber: 7g, Protein: 10g

Cooking Time: 20 minutes
Serves: 4

Instructions:
1. Cook quinoa according to package instructions. Allow to cool slightly.

2. In a large bowl, combine the cooked quinoa, black beans, cucumber, feta cheese, olives, and parsley.
3. In a small bowl, whisk together the lemon juice, olive oil, oregano, salt, and black pepper.
4. Pour the dressing over the quinoa mixture and toss gently to combine.
5. Serve chilled or at room temperature.

Recipe 4:

Tropical Quinoa and Black Bean Salad

Ingredients:
- 1 cup quinoa, rinsed
- 1 (15oz) can black beans, drained and rinsed
- 1 cup diced pineapple
- 1/2 cup diced mango
- 1/4 cup chopped red onion
- 2 tablespoons chopped fresh mint
- 2 tablespoons lime juice
- 1 tablespoon honey
- 1 teaspoon grated lime zest

- 1/4 teaspoon salt

Nutrition (per serving):
Calories: 290, Total Fat: 3g, Saturated Fat: 0g, Sodium: 300mg, Carbohydrates: 54g, Fiber: 9g, Protein: 9g

Cooking Time: 20 minutes
Serves: 4

Instructions:
1. Cook quinoa according to package instructions. Allow to cool slightly.
2. In a large bowl, combine the cooked quinoa, black beans, pineapple, mango, red onion, and mint.
3. In a small bowl, whisk together the lime juice, honey, lime zest, and salt.
4. Pour the dressing over the quinoa mixture and toss gently to combine.
5. Serve chilled or at room temperature.

CHAPTER THREE

Dinner Recipes

- Baked Salmon with Steamed Vegetables

Recipe 1:

Lemon-Herb Baked Salmon with Steamed Broccoli and Carrots

Ingredients:
- 4 (6oz) salmon fillets
- 2 tablespoons olive oil
- 2 tablespoons lemon juice
- 1 teaspoon dried dill
- 1 teaspoon dried parsley
- 1/2 teaspoon salt
- 1/4 teaspoon black pepper
- 2 cups broccoli florets
- 2 cups baby carrots

Nutrition (per serving):
Calories: 350, Total Fat: 18g, Saturated Fat: 3g, Sodium: 450mg, Carbohydrates: 12g, Fiber: 4g, Protein: 37g

Cooking Time: 30 minutes
Serves: 4

Instructions:
1. Preheat the oven to 400°F (200°C).
2. In a small bowl, mix together the olive oil, lemon juice, dill, parsley, salt, and black pepper.
3. Place the salmon fillets in a baking dish and brush the top of each fillet with the lemon-herb mixture.
4. Bake the salmon for 15-18 minutes, or until it flakes easily with a fork.
5. In a steamer basket, steam the broccoli and carrots for 8-10 minutes, or until tender.
6. Serve the baked salmon with the steamed broccoli and carrots.

Recipe 2:

Honey-Mustard Baked Salmon with Steamed Asparagus and Bell Peppers

Ingredients:
- 4 (6oz) salmon fillets
- 2 tablespoons honey
- 2 tablespoons Dijon mustard
- 1 teaspoon garlic powder
- 1/2 teaspoon salt
- 1/4 teaspoon black pepper
- 1 pound asparagus, trimmed
- 1 red bell pepper, sliced

Nutrition (per serving):
Calories: 330, Total Fat: 15g, Saturated Fat: 2g, Sodium: 480mg, Carbohydrates: 13g, Fiber: 3g, Protein: 36g

Cooking Time: 30 minutes
Serves: 4

Instructions:
1. Preheat the oven to 400°F (200°C).

2. In a small bowl, mix together the honey, Dijon mustard, garlic powder, salt, and black pepper.

3. Place the salmon fillets in a baking dish and brush the top of each fillet with the honey-mustard mixture.

4. Bake the salmon for 15-18 minutes, or until it flakes easily with a fork.

5. In a steamer basket, steam the asparagus and bell pepper slices for 8-10 minutes, or until tender.

6. Serve the baked salmon with the steamed asparagus and bell peppers.

Recipe 3:

Teriyaki Baked Salmon with Steamed Bok Choy and Snow Peas

Ingredients:
- 4 (6oz) salmon fillets
- 1/4 cup teriyaki sauce
- 1 tablespoon sesame oil
- 1 teaspoon grated ginger
- 1/4 teaspoon red pepper flakes (optional)

- 2 cups baby bok choy, trimmed
- 1 cup snow peas, trimmed

Nutrition (per serving):
Calories: 340, Total Fat: 16g, Saturated Fat: 3g, Sodium: 550mg, Carbohydrates: 12g, Fiber: 3g, Protein: 37g

Cooking Time: 30 minutes
Serves: 4

Instructions:
1. Preheat the oven to 400°F (200°C).
2. In a small bowl, mix together the teriyaki sauce, sesame oil, grated ginger, and red pepper flakes (if using).
3. Place the salmon fillets in a baking dish and brush the top of each fillet with the teriyaki mixture.
4. Bake the salmon for 15-18 minutes, or until it flakes easily with a fork.
5. In a steamer basket, steam the bok choy and snow peas for 8-10 minutes, or until tender.

6. Serve the baked salmon with the steamed bok choy and snow peas.

Recipe 4:

Parmesan-Crusted Baked Salmon with Steamed Zucchini and Yellow Squash

Ingredients:
- 4 (6oz) salmon fillets
- 1/2 cup grated Parmesan cheese
- 2 tablespoons breadcrumbs
- 1 tablespoon olive oil
- 1 teaspoon dried oregano
- 1/2 teaspoon salt
- 1/4 teaspoon black pepper
- 2 zucchini, sliced
- 2 yellow squash, sliced

Nutrition (per serving):
Calories: 360, Total Fat: 19g, Saturated Fat: 5g, Sodium: 520mg, Carbohydrates: 10g, Fiber: 3g, Protein: 38g

Cooking Time: 30 minutes

Serves: 4

Instructions:
1. Preheat the oven to 400°F (200°C).
2. In a shallow bowl, mix together the Parmesan cheese, breadcrumbs, olive oil, oregano, salt, and black pepper.
3. Place the salmon fillets in a baking dish and press the Parmesan mixture onto the top of each fillet.
4. Bake the salmon for 15-18 minutes, or until the crust is golden brown and the salmon flakes easily with a fork.
5. In a steamer basket, steam the zucchini and yellow squash slices for 8-10 minutes, or until tender.
6. Serve the parmesan-crusted baked salmon with the steamed zucchini and yellow squash.

- Chicken Stir-Fry with Brown Rice

Recipe 1:

Garlic Ginger Chicken Stir-Fry with Brown Rice

Ingredients:
- 1 cup uncooked brown rice
- 1 lb boneless, skinless chicken breasts, cut into 1-inch pieces
- 2 tablespoons vegetable oil
- 3 cloves garlic, minced
- 1 tablespoon grated fresh ginger
- 1 red bell pepper, sliced
- 1 cup broccoli florets
- 1/2 cup sliced mushrooms
- 2 tablespoons soy sauce
- 1 tablespoon rice vinegar
- 1 teaspoon sesame oil
- 1/4 teaspoon red pepper flakes (optional)
- Salt and black pepper to taste

Nutrition (per serving):
Calories: 400, Total Fat: 12g, Saturated Fat: 2g, Sodium: 540mg, Carbohydrates: 42g, Fiber: 4g, Protein: 35g

Cooking Time: 30 minutes
Serves: 4

Instructions:
1. Cook the brown rice according to package instructions.
2. In a large skillet or wok, heat the vegetable oil over high heat.
3. Add the chicken and stir-fry for 4-5 minutes, or until it's no longer pink.
4. Add the garlic, ginger, bell pepper, broccoli, and mushrooms. Stir-fry for another 5-6 minutes, until the vegetables are tender-crisp.
5. Add the soy sauce, rice vinegar, sesame oil, and red pepper flakes (if using). Stir to combine.
6. Serve the chicken stir-fry over the cooked brown rice.

Recipe 2:

Teriyaki Chicken Stir-Fry with Brown Rice

Ingredients:
- 1 cup uncooked brown rice
- 1 lb boneless, skinless chicken breasts, cut into 1-inch pieces
- 2 tablespoons vegetable oil
- 1 cup sliced onion
- 2 cups mixed vegetables (such as snow peas, carrots, and broccoli)
- 1/2 cup teriyaki sauce
- 1 tablespoon cornstarch
- 2 tablespoons water
- Salt and black pepper to taste

Nutrition (per serving):
Calories: 410, Total Fat: 10g, Saturated Fat: 1g, Sodium: 650mg, Carbohydrates: 48g, Fiber: 4g, Protein: 35g

Cooking Time: 30 minutes
Serves: 4

Instructions:
1. Cook the brown rice according to package instructions.

2. In a large skillet or wok, heat the vegetable oil over high heat.
3. Add the chicken and stir-fry for 4-5 minutes, or until it's no longer pink.
4. Add the onion and mixed vegetables. Stir-fry for another 5-6 minutes, until the vegetables are tender-crisp.
5. In a small bowl, whisk together the teriyaki sauce, cornstarch, and water. Pour the mixture into the skillet and bring to a simmer, stirring constantly until the sauce thickens.
6. Serve the teriyaki chicken stir-fry over the cooked brown rice.

Recipe 3:

Thai-Inspired Chicken Stir-Fry with Brown Rice

Ingredients:
- 1 cup uncooked brown rice
- 1 lb boneless, skinless chicken breasts, cut into 1-inch pieces
- 2 tablespoons vegetable oil

- 1 tablespoon Thai red curry paste
- 1 cup sliced mushrooms
- 1 red bell pepper, sliced
- 1 cup sliced cabbage
- 1/2 cup coconut milk
- 2 tablespoons fish sauce
- 1 tablespoon brown sugar
- 1/4 cup chopped fresh cilantro
- Lime wedges for serving

Nutrition (per serving):
Calories: 430, Total Fat: 14g, Saturated Fat: 5g, Sodium: 600mg, Carbohydrates: 44g, Fiber: 4g, Protein: 35g

Cooking Time: 30 minutes
Serves: 4

Instructions:
1. Cook the brown rice according to package instructions.
2. In a large skillet or wok, heat the vegetable oil over high heat.
3. Add the chicken and stir-fry for 4-5 minutes, or until it's no longer pink.

4. Add the Thai red curry paste and stir to coat the chicken.

5. Add the mushrooms, bell pepper, and cabbage. Stir-fry for another 5-6 minutes, until the vegetables are tender-crisp.

6. Pour in the coconut milk, fish sauce, and brown sugar. Bring to a simmer and cook for 2-3 minutes, until the sauce thickens slightly.

7. Serve the Thai-inspired chicken stir-fry over the cooked brown rice, garnished with chopped fresh cilantro and lime wedges.

Recipe 4:

Lemon Pepper Chicken Stir-Fry with Brown Rice

Ingredients:
- 1 cup uncooked brown rice
- 1 lb boneless, skinless chicken breasts, cut into 1-inch pieces
- 2 tablespoons vegetable oil
- 2 teaspoons lemon pepper seasoning

- 1 cup snap peas
- 1 cup sliced zucchini
- 1/2 cup halved cherry tomatoes
- 2 tablespoons lemon juice
- 1 tablespoon soy sauce
- Salt and black pepper to taste

Nutrition (per serving):
Calories: 390, Total Fat: 11g, Saturated Fat: 1g, Sodium: 550mg, Carbohydrates: 44g, Fiber: 4g, Protein: 35g

Cooking Time: 30 minutes
Serves: 4

Instructions:
1. Cook the brown rice according to package instructions.
2. In a large skillet or wok, heat the vegetable oil over high heat.
3. Add the chicken and lemon pepper seasoning. Stir-fry for 4-5 minutes, or until the chicken is no longer pink.

4. Add the snap peas, zucchini, and cherry tomatoes. Stir-fry for another 5-6 minutes, until the vegetables are tender-crisp.
5. Stir in the lemon juice and soy sauce. Season with salt and black pepper to taste.
6. Serve the lemon pepper chicken stir-fry over the cooked brown rice.

- Herb-Crusted Cod with Asparagus

Recipe 1:

Parmesan-Herb Crusted Cod with Roasted Asparagus

Ingredients:
- 4 (6oz) cod fillets
- 1/2 cup panko breadcrumbs
- 1/4 cup grated Parmesan cheese
- 2 tablespoons chopped fresh parsley
- 1 tablespoon chopped fresh thyme
- 1 tablespoon olive oil
- 1/2 teaspoon garlic powder

- 1/4 teaspoon salt
- 1/4 teaspoon black pepper
- 1 lb asparagus, trimmed
- 1 tablespoon olive oil
- 1/4 teaspoon salt
- 1/4 teaspoon black pepper

Nutrition (per serving):
Calories: 310, Total Fat: 12g, Saturated Fat: 3g, Sodium: 480mg, Carbohydrates: 12g, Fiber: 3g, Protein: 36g

Cooking Time: 25 minutes
Serves: 4

Instructions:
1. Preheat the oven to 400°F (200°C).
2. In a shallow bowl, mix together the panko, Parmesan, parsley, thyme, 1 tablespoon olive oil, garlic powder, 1/4 teaspoon salt, and 1/4 teaspoon black pepper.
3. Place the cod fillets in a baking dish and press the breadcrumb mixture onto the top of each fillet.

4. Toss the asparagus with 1 tablespoon olive oil, 1/4 teaspoon salt, and 1/4 teaspoon black pepper. Arrange the asparagus around the cod fillets.

5. Bake for 18-22 minutes, or until the cod is opaque and flakes easily with a fork, and the asparagus is tender-crisp.

6. Serve the parmesan-herb crusted cod with the roasted asparagus.

Recipe 2:

Lemon-Dill Crusted Cod with Steamed Asparagus

Ingredients:
- 4 (6oz) cod fillets
- 1/2 cup panko breadcrumbs
- 2 tablespoons grated lemon zest
- 2 tablespoons chopped fresh dill
- 1 tablespoon olive oil
- 1/4 teaspoon salt
- 1/4 teaspoon black pepper
- 1 lb asparagus, trimmed
- 1/4 cup water

Nutrition (per serving):
Calories: 280, Total Fat: 9g, Saturated Fat: 1g, Sodium: 420mg, Carbohydrates: 11g, Fiber: 3g, Protein: 37g

Cooking Time: 20 minutes
Serves: 4

Instructions:
1. Preheat the oven to 400°F (200°C).
2. In a shallow bowl, mix together the panko, lemon zest, dill, olive oil, 1/4 teaspoon salt, and 1/4 teaspoon black pepper.
3. Place the cod fillets in a baking dish and press the breadcrumb mixture onto the top of each fillet.
4. In a steamer basket, steam the asparagus with 1/4 cup water for 8-10 minutes, or until tender-crisp.
5. Bake the cod for 12-15 minutes, or until it is opaque and flakes easily with a fork.
6. Serve the lemon-dill crusted cod with the steamed asparagus.

Recipe 3:

 Panko-Crusted Cod with Roasted Garlic Asparagus

Ingredients:
- 4 (6oz) cod fillets
- 1 cup panko breadcrumbs
- 2 tablespoons melted butter
- 1 tablespoon chopped fresh parsley
- 1 teaspoon lemon zest
- 1/4 teaspoon salt
- 1/4 teaspoon black pepper
- 1 lb asparagus, trimmed
- 3 cloves garlic, minced
- 2 tablespoons olive oil
- 1/4 teaspoon salt
- 1/4 teaspoon black pepper

Nutrition (per serving):
Calories: 320, Total Fat: 15g, Saturated Fat: 4g, Sodium: 530mg, Carbohydrates: 14g, Fiber: 4g, Protein: 35g

Cooking Time: 25 minutes
Serves: 4

Instructions:
1. Preheat the oven to 400°F (200°C).
2. In a shallow bowl, mix together the panko, melted butter, parsley, lemon zest, 1/4 teaspoon salt, and 1/4 teaspoon black pepper.
3. Place the cod fillets in a baking dish and press the breadcrumb mixture onto the top of each fillet.
4. Toss the asparagus with the minced garlic, 2 tablespoons olive oil, 1/4 teaspoon salt, and 1/4 teaspoon black pepper. Arrange the asparagus around the cod fillets.
5. Bake for 18-22 minutes, or until the cod is opaque and flakes easily with a fork, and the asparagus is tender-crisp.
6. Serve the panko-crusted cod with the roasted garlic asparagus.

Recipe 4:

Herb-Crusted Cod with Lemon-Garlic Asparagus

Ingredients:
- 4 (6oz) cod fillets
- 1/2 cup panko breadcrumbs
- 2 tablespoons grated Parmesan cheese
- 1 tablespoon chopped fresh basil
- 1 tablespoon chopped fresh oregano
- 1 tablespoon olive oil
- 1/4 teaspoon salt
- 1/4 teaspoon black pepper
- 1 lb asparagus, trimmed
- 2 tablespoons olive oil
- 2 cloves garlic, minced
- 1 tablespoon lemon juice
- 1/4 teaspoon salt
- 1/4 teaspoon black pepper

Nutrition (per serving):
Calories: 290, Total Fat: 13g, Saturated Fat: 2g, Sodium: 490mg, Carbohydrates: 12g, Fiber: 4g, Protein: 34g

Cooking Time: 25 minutes

Serves: 4

Instructions:
1. Preheat the oven to 400°F (200°C).
2. In a shallow bowl, mix together the panko, Parmesan, basil, oregano, 1 tablespoon olive oil, 1/4 teaspoon salt, and 1/4 teaspoon black pepper.
3. Place the cod fillets in a baking dish and press the breadcrumb mixture onto the top of each fillet.
4. In a large skillet, heat the 2 tablespoons olive oil over medium heat. Add the minced garlic and sauté for 1 minute.
5. Add the asparagus, lemon juice, 1/4 teaspoon salt, and 1/4 teaspoon black pepper. Sauté for 5-7 minutes, or until the asparagus is tender-crisp.
6. Bake the herb-crusted cod for 18-22 minutes, or until the fish is opaque and flakes easily with a fork.
7. Serve the herb-crusted cod with the lemon-garlic asparagus.

- Low-Sodium Beef Stew

Recipe 1:

Slow Cooker Low-Sodium Beef Stew

Ingredients:
- 1 lb beef stew meat, cut into 1-inch cubes
- 2 cups low-sodium beef broth
- 1 cup diced carrots
- 1 cup diced potatoes
- 1 cup diced celery
- 1 onion, diced
- 2 cloves garlic, minced
- 1 bay leaf
- 1 teaspoon dried thyme
- 1/2 teaspoon black pepper
- 1/4 teaspoon salt

Nutrition (per serving):
Calories: 270, Total Fat: 8g, Saturated Fat: 3g, Sodium: 240mg, Carbohydrates: 18g, Fiber: 3g, Protein: 27g

Cooking Time: 6-8 hours (in slow cooker)
Serves: 4

Instructions:
1. Place the beef stew meat, low-sodium beef broth, carrots, potatoes, celery, onion, garlic, bay leaf, thyme, black pepper, and salt in a slow cooker.
2. Cover and cook on low for 6-8 hours, or until the beef and vegetables are tender.
3. Remove the bay leaf before serving.
4. Serve the low-sodium beef stew.

Recipe 2:

One-Pot Low-Sodium Beef Stew

Ingredients:
- 1 lb beef stew meat, cut into 1-inch cubes
- 2 cups low-sodium beef broth
- 1 cup diced tomatoes (no-salt-added)
- 1 cup frozen peas
- 1 cup diced potatoes
- 1/2 cup diced onion
- 2 cloves garlic, minced

- 1 teaspoon dried oregano
- 1/2 teaspoon black pepper
- 1/4 teaspoon salt

Nutrition (per serving):
Calories: 260, Total Fat: 7g, Saturated Fat: 2g, Sodium: 220mg, Carbohydrates: 20g, Fiber: 4g, Protein: 26g

Cooking Time: 45 minutes
Serves: 4

Instructions:
1. In a large pot or Dutch oven, brown the beef stew meat over medium-high heat.
2. Add the low-sodium beef broth, diced tomatoes, frozen peas, potatoes, onion, garlic, oregano, black pepper, and salt.
3. Bring the stew to a boil, then reduce the heat and simmer for 30-35 minutes, or until the beef and vegetables are tender.
4. Serve the low-sodium beef stew.

Recipe 3:

Instant Pot Low-Sodium Beef Stew

Ingredients:
- 1 lb beef stew meat, cut into 1-inch cubes
- 1 cup low-sodium beef broth
- 1 cup diced carrots
- 1 cup diced celery
- 1 cup diced potatoes
- 1/2 cup diced onion
- 2 cloves garlic, minced
- 1 bay leaf
- 1 teaspoon dried thyme
- 1/2 teaspoon black pepper
- 1/4 teaspoon salt

Nutrition (per serving):
Calories: 280, Total Fat: 8g, Saturated Fat: 3g, Sodium: 230mg, Carbohydrates: 19g, Fiber: 3g, Protein: 28g

Cooking Time: 30 minutes (in Instant Pot)
Serves: 4

Instructions:

1. Place the beef stew meat, low-sodium beef broth, carrots, celery, potatoes, onion, garlic, bay leaf, thyme, black pepper, and salt in an Instant Pot.
2. Close the lid and set the Instant Pot to the "Stew/Meat" function for 30 minutes.
3. Once the cooking time is up, allow the pressure to release naturally for 10 minutes, then release the remaining pressure.
4. Remove the bay leaf before serving.
5. Serve the low-sodium beef stew.

Recipe 4:

Oven-Baked Low-Sodium Beef Stew

Ingredients:
- 1 lb beef stew meat, cut into 1-inch cubes
- 2 cups low-sodium beef broth
- 1 cup diced sweet potatoes
- 1 cup diced butternut squash
- 1/2 cup diced onion
- 2 cloves garlic, minced
- 1 teaspoon dried rosemary

- 1/2 teaspoon black pepper
- 1/4 teaspoon salt

Nutrition (per serving):
Calories: 290, Total Fat: 8g, Saturated Fat: 3g, Sodium: 240mg, Carbohydrates: 21g, Fiber: 4g, Protein: 29g

Cooking Time: 1 hour 30 minutes
Serves: 4

Instructions:
1. Preheat the oven to 325°F (165°C).
2. In a large oven-safe pot or Dutch oven, combine the beef stew meat, low-sodium beef broth, sweet potatoes, butternut squash, onion, garlic, rosemary, black pepper, and salt.
3. Cover the pot and bake for 1 hour 30 minutes, or until the beef and vegetables are tender.
4. Serve the low-sodium beef stew.

Living with kidney disease can present unique dietary challenges, but with the right knowledge and guidance, you can take control of your health and nourish your body with the essential foods it needs. The comprehensive food lists we've provided offer a roadmap to navigating the complexities of kidney-friendly eating, empowering you to make informed choices that support your overall well-being.

By incorporating these renal-friendly ingredients into your meals, you can help manage symptoms, slow disease progression, and maintain optimal kidney function. From low-sodium whole grains and lean proteins to potassium-rich fruits and vegetables, these carefully curated lists ensure you have the tools to create delicious and nutritious dishes that cater to your specific dietary needs.

Remember, managing kidney disease is a journey, and the path forward may require patience, experimentation, and a willingness to adapt. But with this essential guide by your side, you can navigate the complexities with confidence, nourishing your body and taking proactive steps towards improved kidney health. Embark on this culinary adventure with a renewed sense of purpose, and let these recipes and recommendations be your guide to a healthier, more fulfilling life.

www.ingramcontent.com/pod-product-compliance
Lightning Source LLC
Chambersburg PA
CBHW050821250726
48653CB00006B/2349